GUIDE AND NUITRITION FOR PREGNANCY

COMPLETE DIET

Jessica C. Nevberry

Contents

Chapter One

Foreword

Human nutrition has been sad lately, besieged from one side by a relentless publicity in the service of a formidable industry, and the other by a legion of pseudo-experts who propose diets to which more capricious in books that sometimes top the bestseller lists (but not for long time, because soon a new diet appears that says the opposite, and They also follow her in Hollywood!). The Mediterranean diet of which we so much we were proud he on Frank recoil in view of the avalanche from appetizers salty, fatty frozen and dairy desserts. The heavy dishes that were previously reserved for very few celebrations now occupy our tables almost daily; many let the water run that they should not drink, because they prefer to drink anything else, better with sugar, and some seem to believe that a food cannot be healthy, what is said to be healthy, if our grandparents already ate it or if it doesn't come from some distant country or from some ancient culture.

It is therefore increasingly convenient to have a nutritionist trust What July basult, what bases their recommendations on data scientists; what no us "regenerate", neither us «detoxifies», neither even us "energizes"; that does not promise health without blemish, happiness without guilt, effortless thinness or eternal life.

The diet of pregnant and lactating mothers should basically be normal. The same diet fury what should to enjoy everything the world, men's and women, with children or without children, but from which we have been moving away. No

I know treats, well, from do a "sacrifice" during some months for later go back to eating chips and soft drinks, but to stop sacrificing ourselves, to stop sacrifice our health on the altar of fashion and advertising, and learn to eat normally for the rest of our lives. Because what really goes to influence the long-term health of our children is not what we have eaten during pregnancy (which influences only a little) nor what we eat during the lactation (what no influences almost nothing), otherwise the habits what will acquire by eating at our side for the next twenty years or more. Our way of eating no longer affects only us; have also the responsibility of being a good role model for our children. The feeding healthy the form foods healthy, no «nutrients healthy»

What consumers, we went out winning when we think plus on terms from foods what from nutrients. By the contrary, the Business get top results Yes they speak from nutrients on place from, simply, foods.

J UANJO C ACERES, Consumption smart

TO SEA THE PLOT PLUS WHAT THE OUTCOME

In the next chapters I will focus fully on the particularities of the nutrition of pregnant or breastfeeding women. However, I think that before it is necessary to describe the characteristics that it has (and that it does not have) a healthy diet. In case it crosses your mind to skip this chapter, I remember it what it says the saying: "No let way by take sidewalk, what you think you overtake but you surround ». This other one also comes in handy: «Dress me slowly, what I have rush", what on tongue English is common hear on is other shape: « More have done, less speed » ("TO plus rush, less speed"). Can what no tea persuade the sayings by that from "people proverbs, lying people. If I answered you with "people of proverbs, people of truths", possibly it would not convince you either, and that is why I have used, to title this section, the verse "love the plot more than the outcome" of the great singer-songwriter (and doctor) George Drexler.

Let's go well with the plot.

Chapter Two

NO GIVES SAME THE DAY WHAT FOLLOW

Health, at all stages of the life cycle (such as pregnancy and lactation), no depends so much the doctor, the number from drugs, from "medicinal plants" or "fat burners" that we take, much less the number from regimens dietary miraculous, "depurative" and quirky what let's do, otherwise from a word call "diet", what comes from the Greek term diaita . For the Greeks, diet referred to regulation of life habits in general, including food. Thus, according to this healthy and ancestral perspective, we cannot ignore that tobacco, poor diet, physical inactivity and alcohol cause the higher part from the deaths on our country, neither what the bad Habits are going global. The rapid urbanization and globalization of unhealthy lifestyles, among other reasons, are determining our health," said Dr. Margaret Chan, director of general of the World Organization for Health (WHO).

We have proof of this in a study that followed up from 2,000 males during 35 years, on the I know defined, before from begin, five related items with health:

No to smoke.

Maintain a healthy weight (learn more in Chapter 6).

Consume more than three daily servings of fruits and vegetables (they pointed out low, because in reality it is convenient for us adults to take more than five servings/day).

To practice exercise from shape regular.

Drink little bit alcohol.

The research, pickup on the edition from December by PLoS One, found that less than 1 percent of volunteers met all five aforementioned parameters. The 35-year follow-up also showed that the number from individuals whose habits from Health they were good ones I was "Stagnant". The data is bleak enough for those of us who we dedicate ourselves to health, let it be as impossible. Dr. Wendy Levinson published in 2001 (Annals of Internal Medicine) another equally discouraging: only 20 percent of patients seeking medical services are willing to make sustained changes in their lifestyle. But I am not one of those who throw in the towel just like that, but one of those who think that constancy all the reach, so that there I go.

The confluence from a feeding healthy (or, better saying, "no unhealthy"), the routine practice of physical activity and avoiding smoking can prevent as many as 90 percent of type II diabetes, 80 percent of the diseases the heart, the 70 percent from the spills cerebral and about the 70 percent from the cancers. Yes us we center on the nutrition, the WHO assures that "improving nutrition could be the most important isolate for disease reduction. The phrase appears in his book Food and Health in Europe: a New Basis for Action. In it we read that 8 out of 10 diseases that cause us to lose «years of life healthy" have a component nutritional accused or "very accused".

For the WHO, of the 10 risks that most harm health, 6 are directly related to food, and cause 40 percent of the deaths.

I'll bet you've read or heard dozens of times that the fruits and vegetables are healthy, although I

don't know if you are aware of the magnitude of the issue: 1.7 million deaths could be prevented every year Yes we would take enough amount from these foods, according the WHO.

How about? But wait, there is more: a magnificent study carried out conducted by Reiss and colleagues in December 2012 (Food and Chemical Toxicology) revealed that if half the American population took a ration plus every day from fruit and vegetables I know could avoid 20,000 cancer cases each year. They also evaluated whether the pesticides used on the culture from these foods supposed a trouble, for conclude what "Consumers should not be concerned about the risks of breast cancer consume conventionally grown fruits and vegetables.

No to know detect Yes something on you style from lifetime tea generate problems. I know they need ideas very simple what no I know they teach on the schools. This is the tragedy.

I would also like to wake the legislators out of their lethargy so that restrict the cooking pot to Pressure from the advertising from food unhealthy directed children (very intelligent and very well calculated, like a "smart" missile) and that prohibit alienating advertising (direct, indirect or covert) of the alcohol. I do not ask for it on my own, it was proposed by the WHO in 2010 in its «Report on the global situation of non-communicable diseases". I'll talk about it later, but, first, a review of the concept of "eating everything". Feeding and fertility

Yes no we develop our faculties critics we stayed defenseless against the arguments and harangues of people without good intention.

T HOMAS Gilovich, convinced but wrong, Barcelona, A thousand reasons, 2009.

OBSERVATIONS IMPORTANT

If you and your partner are trying to conceive a child, the most important thing is that make love often (with each other and without protection, of course). It's a truism, I know, but in many cases the supposed lack of Fertility is nothing more than a low frequency of sexual intercourse. It is also crucial that if you smoke, you stop as soon as possible, both. It is something that usually works better with medical help. It is convenient that avoid both alcoholic beverages (in the case of women, the ideal is not drink neither gout from alcohol) what the sedentary lifestyle or a diet unbalanced, and what no consume drugs, accessories food or "floors medicines" without adequate medical advice. TO PURCHASE CRITERION

After these few initial recommendations, which summarize the most important of this chapter, I would like to clarify that one of the objectives that I pursue with this book is that you don't let your guard down at any time, because in the ground from the feeding human the amount from tricksters is infinite and I know expand, What the universe. From there the appointment the psychologist Thomas Gilovich who heads this chapter and who urges us to develop "our critical faculties. I have always believed that we should be critical, but now I know that, in addition, we must "acquire judgment." I explain.

A few months ago, my wife and I savored a conversation with Joan Artigal, a magnificent teacher of one of our daughters. In certain moment, I explained to him that in the book No More Diet I had included a reflection of which he was very proud: «Common sense is fine, but is better yet the sense critical".

Joan I I'm listening, smiled and said: "Great, July. I thought it same make some years". When talks an intelligent person it is better not to interrupt him, so my wife and I we wait to what continue speaking, knowing what I know was coming something important. «Today I believe that before resorting to the critical spirit it is necessary gain judgment." That lapidary «acquire criterion", to what we answered to the unison with a "have all the reason, John." The lines what follow pretend, precisely, contribute something from "criterion". The zinc gets better the fertility?

This brings us to zinc and the weak points of the Regulation. Because if we type on the box from search from bliss Web words What " fertility ", " reproduction ", « reproductive system » or others Similar we see what the EFSA has indeed approved a health claim in relation to fertility. Is the following: "The zinc contributes to a fertility and reproduction normal". Is certain. So certain what yes us they would say what "Breathe contributes to a fertility and reproduction normal". Something very different to "Breathing more often will improve your fertility" or "Take more zinc it will make your fertility better."

I say this because the scientific opinion that approves the declaration for the zinc indicates that the evidence reviewed does not establish that in the population general from the Union European exist intakes inadequate from zinc what drive to a deterioration from the fertility. Even though outside certain what we were ingesting little zinc with the diet, it is not a situation that lead to reproductive problems. If you give a malnourished woman a diet delicious on zinc, will increase the possibilities from what I know stay pregnant... even though maybe no be Thank you to saying mineral, otherwise to the confluence of other necessary factors (a man who is neither malnourished nor infertile) with others aspects nutritional (Energy, acids fatty, proteins, vitamins, etc).

In 2012, the Ministry of Health, Social Services and Equality, through of the Spanish Agency for Consumer Affairs, Food Safety and Nutrition, public the first poll national from intake dietetics Spanish, named ENIDE. In it we read that "zinc deficiency due to is rare", that "the functional consequences of intakes low from zinc on the adult is it so little bit studied» and, no less importantly, that taking too much zinc "can alter the metabolism of copper, the immune response and blood cells.

Since it is possible (and legal) for you to find food or supplements food what put on letters capital letters what «contains zinc, what contributes to normal fertility and reproduction", my advice is the next: do not fall for their traps and do not spend your money on false promises. Take a food supplement, except for express medical indication, it can be more harmful than beneficial. ACID FOLIC, SALT IODINE AND VITAMIN B12

I will expand more fully on folic acid and iodized salt in the next chapter (see Folic Acid and Iodine in Chapter 3), now so I will just say that taking a daily supplement containing 400 micrograms (no milligrams) from acid folic three months before from the conception contributes to the growth of maternal tissue in pregnancy and prevents called "neural tube defects", a series of (serious) problems of the nervous system of the fetus. An investigation collected in the July issue of 2014 of the scientific journal Obstetrics and Gynecology adds a minor risk of miscarriage among women taking this supplement.

As for iodine, take a pinch of iodized salt (which we should not confused with "sea salt", "flower of salt", "Maldon salt", or Menorca salt, Cristina Island, the Himalayas or any other point on the planet) is a good way from cover our requirements from East nutrient crucial for health. The recommendation applies to the whole of society, not just to pregnant women, but in them it is especially important, since a deficit moderate from iodine during the pregnancy I know ha related with a higher incidence from problems gestational and even with the quotient intellectual the baby. So much the recommendation from consume acid folic what that of taking iodized salt is issued today by any entity involved in health or in nutrition.

Special mention deserves vitamin B12 in vegetarian people because the deficiency of this vitamin, common in this group, is related with infertility and with recurrent fetal loss 5. If you follow a diet vegetarian, I advise you to review the section that I dedicate to this pattern feeding in chapter 8.

Chapter Three

SYNDROME THE OVARY POLYCYSTIC

I devote a section to East syndrome, which affects a significant number of women (between 6% and 21%, more so if they are overweight), and which creates challenges for what I know produces a successful pregnancy (menstrual dysfunctions, infertility or increased risk of complications in gestation). WEIGHT LOSS OR ADDITIONAL WEIGHT PRIOR TO PREGNANCY

Obesity may affect reproductive rates. Chapter 6 delves more into this subject. In these few lines, I want to emphasize that while there is never a good time to "make diet" (that is, to adhere to a restrictive regimen and stray from a healthy eating pattern), it is especially unwise prior to pregnancy, immediately following childbirth, and (especially) during the nine months of pregnancy. When someone casually proposes a "diet," whether it's to lose weight, gain muscle, or produce more milk, enquire about its efficacy and safety. If he does not provide them to you (in writing) or if the ones he does provide are delicate, such as a Chinese vase, remind him of the following line by Christopher Hitchens: "Whatever may be claimed without proof can also be denied without evidence." ADDITIONAL IMPORTANT IMPORTANT IMPORTANT HOW DOES IT AFFECT FERTILITY?

Is there anything that may help you become more fertile? Naturally, there is, which is why facilities for assisted reproduction exist. If you choose to visit a private facility (which must be regulated and certified by the Ministry of Health), keep in mind that no tea "guarantees" results and that treatment will not often be inexpensive. However, is it possible to work remotely? We have a better understanding of what actions should be taken to avoid jeopardizing fertility and what actions should be taken to enhance it. Antoine de Saint-Exupéry once said, in the context of a renowned remark on technical and aeronautical advancement, that "Perfection seems to be attained not when there is nothing more to add, but when there is nothing more to repress." I'll devote the following lines to it: to attempt to eliminate any probable flaws. Lifestyle characterized by inactivity

Sedentary lifestyles, as I am aware, are also associated with a high mortality rate, namely 5.3 million fatalities every year. The data comes from a thorough investigation published in the July 2012 edition of the Lancet in which Lee et al. concluded that inactivity contributes to roughly as many premature deaths as smoking. Even if our bodies do not react well to inactivity, we ignore their warnings and illnesses, as more than 40% of people in Spain consider themselves to be "inactive" in their spare time.

Is there a link between chair abuse and fertility? If that is the case, Sharpe and Franks conducted an experiment in October 2002 in the scientific journal Nature Cell Biology demonstrating that a sedentary lifestyle has a significant impact on both women and men's fertility. According to some, athletes' sperm deteriorates as a result of physical activity. That is not what Dr. Lidia Minguez-Alarcon (from Murcia's Faculty of Medicine) and her colleagues noticed in their investigation, which included the July 2014 edition of the periodical Fertility and Sterility. On he elaborated on what "physical exercise is not harmful to testicular function." A few years back, a cycle of news reported about how extreme exercise causes women to become infertile. He quickly uncovered the scam using the Health NHS Choices webpage, as I previously said.

Yes, we are aware of the ways in which a sedentary lifestyle might affect fertility directly (by impairing sperm quality or interfering with ovulation) or indirectly. A possible contribution is as follows: when we are sedentary, our condition deteriorates, which reduces our chances of having sex with our spouse. Another reason for a sedentary lifestyle is that it raises the risk of obesity, which has a detrimental effect on reproductive function. Human diet "Body weight and nutritional condition are intrinsically linked to reproductive function." This appointment was published in December 2007's Current Opinion in Endocrinology, Diabetes, and Obesity. I have already discussed the necessity of maintaining a healthy weight and avoiding unhealthy behaviors in order to avoid obesity. Now would want to make it very clear what No one diet will boost our fertility rates or the quality of our eggs or sperm when consumed in isolation. Yes, a healthy eating pattern will result in the medium or long term.

We should be suspicious of diets labeled with surnames such as "alkaline," "dissociated," "from the zone," "the sanguine group," "flash," Paleolithic "Pronokal," or "Ayurvedic." Additionally, macrobiotics, which I explain while discussing iodine in Chapter 4 (Algae and Iodine). The worst are often identified by a very legitimate surname such as Atkins, Dukan, Montignac, or Planas. Chronically poor diet results in amenorrhea (absence of menstruation), which clearly has a detrimental effect on fertility. Recently, I've developed a suspicion for those who promote the Mediterranean diet, because they almost always overlook the fact that wine, which is included in the definition of said diet (check it out in the RAE's dictionary if you don't believe me), is an alcoholic beverage and thus increases the risk of developing a variety of disorders and diseases.

As I previously stated, there is never a good time to follow a low-calorie diet, but now is a better time than ever, and not just because of the "Rebound effect," but also because if you are already pregnant (a high proportion of pregnancies occur without the future mom being aware of it), the "diet" may harm the unborn child. If a fetus does not get an enough supply of energy and nutrients throughout its essential early stages of development, their organs may not form properly (ex: brain).

What's already in position I've outlined the characteristics of a diet frenzy (see What is a healthy diet?). I already follow it, as I eat a very varied and "everything" (sic) diet (see chapter 1), so I will not elaborate further on this point, although I want to emphasize that adopting both a good (or bad) feeding scheme and a good (or evil) lifestyle throughout one's life has an effect on the quality of the ovules and sperm. Afeiche and partners offered an example in the journal Journal of Nutrition's July 2014 issue. They noticed that when processed meat consumption increased, the spermatozoa's shape deteriorated and their number decreased. MULTIPLICITY OF PREGNANCY

Following this nutritional examination that you will get during your pregnancy, I feel compelled to devote nail "prayers" to multiple pregnancies, which are increasing in frequency as a result of the growing use of assisted reproductive procedures. It will not be difficult, as a thorough scientific study titled "Nutritional recommendations to enhance pregnancy outcomes in multiple pregnancies." Dr. Celia K. Ballard organized the symposium in June 2011. His assessment of whether or not these ladies need a calorie-dense diet:

Increasing weight growth artificially may not be beneficial and may be distressing for the mother. It may also lead to long-term health concerns as a result of the excess weight.

The article discussed not just the importance of calories in pregnancy, but also the nutrients stated previously: carbs, proteins, lipids (especially Omega 3), vitamins, and minerals. They concluded that it is unclear if providing a particular diet or nutritional advise to women who have numerous pregnancies "can do more benefit than harm." Not unexpectedly, NICE advises that health professionals provide twins or triplets pregnant women "the same advice on nutritional supplements, food, and lifestyle» as the rest of the pregnant women.

E N RESUME

Except for the numbered assumptions, no effort by pregnant Spanish women to drink more water than their thirst dictates, to consume more calories than their appetite dictates (due to "eating for two"), or to consume more protein than they already do is justified (because of the "meat makes meat").

Yes, it seems appropriate to reduce the intake of highly processed foods rich in fats and sugars. Supplementing certain nutrients during pregnancy may expose the fetus to risk at certain concentrations, which should be carefully balanced by a professional sanitary. Is the case, on everything, of vitamins A, D and E, but also of the "candida" vitamin C and of the famous omega-3, especially if they come in capsules of oil of fish liver?

By other part, no make lack (and no is recommendable) cram to the pregnant with calories, proteins, "omega tresses" or multivitamins chachis pirulis, nor is it that we take on our own and risk nutritional supplements (and even less drugs) not prescribed by a professional sanitary accredited. On the following chapter you will understand (or so I hope) that is not interested in doing it with dietary supplements either-nutritional supplements, "medicinal" herbs or "healing" teas or granules of sugar (they call them "homeopathic") (they call them "homeopathic").

We have seen that, as the nutritional demands of the pregnant, other mechanisms such as appetite, thirst or the rate of absorption of the nutrients ingested I know adapt and allow what, on general, everything flow without setbacks forever what the feeding be minimally balanced. The exceptions to be aware of are:

Fiber: To meet the fiber requirements during pregnancy, we should prioritize foods that are minimally processed vegetables (and that have fewer superfluous products in the pantry and refrigerator).

Folic Acid and Folate: Abundant and Strong Evidence Supports Usefulness to supplement pregnant women with 400 micrograms each day of acid folic acid (in addition to consuming fruits and vegetables daily), during a minimum one month before pregnancy and up to three months after conception. On certain cases (valued by a doctor) I know recommend higher doses of this vitamin.

Iodine: I know recommends consume every day a pinch from Salt iodized (what is not synonymous with "sea salt") (what is not synonymous with "sea salt"). The Ministry of Health suggests the supplementation pharmacological during all the gestation with 200 micrograms of iodine (as potassium iodide) in all women who take less than 2 grams of iodized salt and less than three servings of milk and derivatives dairy products (what they contribute iodine because I know It includes at the moment on the feeding from the cows -Some studies show what the milk "ecological" no would a good source from iodine\s—) . Algae usually have a lot of iodine (and in a concentration very variable), so its consumption must be exceptional, in its case.

Iron: the WHO has recommended in 2014 to supplement pregnant women with iron, although in Spain the prescription of this mineral is made only under criterion doctor individualized (something what have a lot sense) (something what have a lot sense).

Vitamin B12: there are folic acid preparations that contain a little B12 (the order from two micrograms), a practice what contributes Benefits and that does not expose us to any danger. Pregnant or lactating vegetarians should be aware of the paramount importance of this vitamin in health maternal and child\s8. There are something plus what I would like what remember all woman pregnant: adopt a good Pattern from feeding be better for mother and child what rely on the powers of isolated nutrients, whether they come from food or from tablets. If during pregnancy we continue with the bad habits that characterize, no we will arrive to make up for the situation by plus "little help" that we take I end with a sentence that you will have heard from your mother more than once and whose origin dates back to the dawn of the history of man: "It is not the cleanest who cleans the most, but the one who dirties the least". Or put in other words: in the "room" of pregnancy there is less space, from a sanitary point of view, for "dirt" and carelessness that inevitably lead to bad habits.

4

Risks nutritional during the pregnancy

To often, it unique what lack is information, and no an amazing molecule novelty.

B IN GOLDACRE, Bad science

As dietitians-nutritionists, we are not only interested in nutrients, but also certain substances no nutritious presents on foods, beverages or accessories food, such What caffeine, alcohol, additives, microorganisms, allergens or environmental contaminants. But what interest us does not mean we are obsessed. No need to get to extreme reflected by the humorist El Perich on February 27, 1992 in El Newspaper. He drew a vignette showing a married couple sitting at the table pronouncing these words before eating: "Bless Lord - and on everything analyze— the food what we are going to consume. Amen".

On everything case, the two risks nutritional plus important on the pregnancy 1, alcohol and tobacco are no joke. Does tobacco escape? In the dietary field? Well no. There are two reasons. The first is that smoking negatively affects the metabolism of various nutrients, such as acid folic, crucial for the correct training the tube neural the fetus. AND the second is that the word 'diet', as I have already explained (I don't care repeat it) comes from the Greek term diaita, which encompasses any habit of health. TO FOOD POTENTIALLY ALLERGENICS

Until 2009, many healthy pregnant (and lactating) women were recommended what no they will take foods potentially allergens (eg: walnuts or peanuts) (eg: walnuts or peanuts). The advice was more usual in case pregnant women they had a risk potential from give to light to a child with allergy food (Yes already they had dice to light to a child with some class from allergy, let's put by case). However, an extensive review changed this view. I know published in December 2010 in the Journal of Allergy and Clinical Immunology and conducted by a panel of experts from the National Institute of Allergy and Infectious Diseases of the United States (NIAID, in its acronym in English) (NIAID, in its acronym in English). Nowadays, all the serious guides that deal with the diet of the pregnant woman discourage the mother from avoiding foods specifically in order to prevent food allergies.

Moreover, there are studies what suggest what Yes the mother consume possible allergens presents on common foods could even prevent food allergy in the baby, although the data on this is inconclusive.

E N RESUME

If you've made it this far, thanks for your patience. I hope you understand that I have to expand to justify statements as unusual as some of which I summarize in the following fourteen points:

Tobacco, marijuana, cocaine and alcohol should be avoided in pregnancy (and in any other situation and age, of course). Beer "without" can have up to 1 percent alcohol, and there are studies that indicate that the 0.0 percent can actually contain up to 1.8 percent .

Food safety is always important, but at this stage is plus. TO the advice usual (see Seat belt food , in chapter 4) we must add that it is not convenient that pregnant women consume pâté (including vegetable pâtés), cheeses soft, such as camembert, feta, brie, blue cheeses, or fresh cheese, unless the labels say they are pasteurized. You should not touch rodents, even pets, until the baby is born.

Yes the pregnant woman no ha past a disease named "toxoplasmosis" before pregnancy, if the meat your cat eats does not is cooked and Yes East no it lives exclusively on his flat, is better what avoid a Contact near with he and what no wipe the animal excrement (or do it with gloves and a mask). It is also justified to freeze raw delicatessen (eg ham), 22 degrees below zero for about ten days before consuming it... in case to do it.

Eating more than three to four servings of fish a week can suppose ingest too mercury. The Ministry from Health Spanish recommended on 2011 to the women pregnant or what can be, as well as lactating women, avoid eating the species most contaminated with mercury (swordfish, shark, bluefin tuna — Thunnus thynnus – large species, normally eaten fresh or frozen and filleted—and pike). The Review, Study and positioning from the Association Spanish from Dieticians- Nutritionists I consider justified do extensible are recommendations to all canned tuna.

The liver contains a lot vitamin TO, by it what is discouraged in this stage.

Yes tea they like the walnuts from Brazil, no take plus from six units daily. Do it increases the risk from suffer "toxicity by selenium" or seleniosis.

The algae have a lofty contents on iodine. How many less, better.

I know discourages drink energy drinks" (type Net Bull).

No is Clear Yes is sure drink plus from 200 milligrams from caffeine/day (the Table 5 details excuse me avoid overcome this figure).

We have little information on the safety of infusions in pregnant. It is worth not exceeding four cups a day in this stage, and ask a health professional when in doubt as to whether an infusion or herbal tea is or is not safe.

Few drugs are safe in pregnancy. Should be used at least possible and then from what a doctor is valued the relationship risk/benefit.

Phytotherapy is not recommended during pregnancy.

Drink to daily Many foods what contain a sweetener called stevia (E-960) can mean exceeding the margins safety of this additive.

No is justified what the pregnant avoid foods potentially allergenic (unless the mother has an allergy food, of course).

5 Problems related with the nutrition from the pregnant

Nutrition is an essential part of health and medicine, and Nutrition science is a vibrant research program and successful. However, nutrition is also a common excuse for the commercialization from pseudoscience medical doubtful and harmful. Doctor S TEVEN N OVELLA

Chapter Four

SOME WORDS PLUS ON THE "FLOORS MEDICINAL»

Nine months give for many doubts, many myths and many scams, about especially when there are problems like some that I detail in this chapter. Because those doubts can lead us down the wrong path, I am going to start by following the thread of something that I commented at the end of the previous one chapter: the risk of relying on so-called «alternative medicine» (the one that when it demonstrates its efficacy and safety it ceases to be an alternative) and, in especially in "herbal supplements". And there are paths that are better no drink for avoid stumbles the pregnant looking for help Yes I know find well, but plus yet when have inconvenience, and is it so willing to spend your money, your time and your trust (which also wears away) on therapies, even though be alternatives. On Many cases, only Yes They are alternatives. The promoters from the therapies alternatives explain stuff sensible, but usually deck them out with quackery dangerous. Yes a freeway is well paved, but contains every 200 meters a long row of tacks, better to avoid it, I think.

From there what some collective appeal, for step land firm, to the called "precautionary principle": if a proposal could pose a risk to the Health, no compensated by the Benefits what contributes, should to put on quarantine. In many of the conditions described in this chapter (I would say than in all of them), we are going to find alternative proposals with little substance, but the most worrying, in my opinion, is the so-called "phytotherapy". I am going to allow me be reiterative with respect to it already commented on the subsection «the "naturalness" of the "medicinal plants" of the previous chapter, because until the 55 percent from the pregnant uses these treatments and because his Utilization is greatest during the first trimester of pregnancy (when the woman tends to have more bothersome symptoms), just when they are most dangerous, already what is a period critic of the development of fetal organs.

We often unthinkingly accept that such products, widely disseminated on web pages or magazines (paid for by companies that sell dietary-nutritional supplements), are safe and harmless. However, scientific rigor, which must be applied to any substance ingested by a pregnant woman, reveals that: The ingredients assets from the extracts from floors they are substances drug-like chemicals.

The "floors medicinal» present the same potential from cause serious adverse effects than other medicines.

Independent analyzes reveal that herbal remedies are not always they contain it what declares the hashtag, when they carry (to times I know they buy on the herbalism, or is it so evil tagged or no have hashtag).

Some accessories herbal they contain quantities from metals potentially toxic heavy.

No there are studies scientists rigorous on the security from are substances.

As you can see, they are not exactly the eighth earthly wonder. That's why to the sanitary us cost understand by what many pregnant women what is it so enduring very bothersome symptoms are

afraid to take a drug prescribed by his doctor 1 , but no doubt on go to the «remedies natural," such as plant-based treatments (blue cohosh, lemon balm, aloe vera, hellebore, tragacanth, ginseng, etc). If you don't want to do guinea pig in full gestation, it is best not to resort to them. Various members the centers for disease Control and Prevention, a from the greater authorities on the ambit sanitary, published on May from 2010 a research on the magazine American Journal of obstetrics and Gynecology , titled "Use from herbs before and during the pregnancy". His "opinion" was as follows:

Healthcare professionals should routinely ask their patients if they use products plant-based and must educate them to understand that we know very little about the risk that supposed use these products.

There is a strong critical current towards medicalization 2 (with which I take communion one hundred percent), but there is not the same disposition towards therapies alternatives, what as well medicalize. Everyone we should have an attitude plus cautious, no self-medicate so much (be with drugs or with "natural supplements"), not believing that there is a magic pill for each symptom and, of course, improve our habits. That said, what if you have not yet classified me as persona non grata, in the following lines I will board briefly some from the problems plus frequent on is stage, which are related to food. In case of any doubt about the appearance of a symptom during your pregnancy, go to the doctor. If a doctor does not convince you, change your doctor. It is true that there are professionals sanitary incompetent (there are morning song on everyone the corners the planet) but that does not mean that current medicine is invalid. On certain cases from preeclampsia or from diabetes gestational, by place two examples, the role of medicine is decisive.

Chapter Five

SIMTOMS GASTROINTESTINAL

Gastrointestinal symptoms are no joke: nausea and vomiting affect to plus from the half from the women pregnant. The constipation, meanwhile, affects 1 in 4, while 2 in 3 pregnant women suffer from heartburn ("heartburn").

The sickness and the vomiting no forever they are a bad sign

In most cases, nausea and vomiting occur between weeks 4 and 7 after the latest period menstrual, and almost forever refer Come in weeks 16 and 20 of gestation. Between 5 and 10 percent of women, who now is little bit, will suffer East discomfort plus there from the week 22 and, unfortunately, there will be women who feel bad until delivery. Usually call it "morning sickness", but the truth is that less than 2 percent of Women have these symptoms only in the morning. Some women look unable to maintain their work activities and even the normal ones of the daily life.

Well, there is a fact that, although it does not improve the symptoms of a pregnant woman, can reassure her, on everything Yes think what his discomfort is a bad omen: unless they are severe (it is not usual), these symptoms are consistently associated with a greater chance that a healthy baby is born. This was verified, among others, by Dr. Ronna L. Chan and their collaborators on November from 2010 on the magazine man Playback.

There are several hypotheses that could explain why this happens:

The symptom appear when I know places on March the framework hormone necessary for a good pregnancy. This framework causes unpleasant symptoms, so their appearance would be proof that the pregnancy is on a good course.

The discomfort prevents what the mother ingest an excess from calories. It would prevent excessive, potentially harmful weight gain.

It could be that smoking or drinking alcohol (or other harmful habits that are relate with a higher risk from abortion) reduce the symptom gastric. Thus, the absence of such symptoms would be associated with the fact that smoking or drinking, two habits that increase the risks for the fetus, and that could explain why women without symptoms have pregnancies less successful.

Women with these symptoms receive more family and social support, which may exert a protective effect on the developing fetus.

Surely the explanation will be in a combination of the above possibilities. I hope you understand that we are dealing with a factor that must be taken into account among the many that determine

the success of a pregnancy. I explain it so you don't get scared if you are pregnant but not you suffer symptom any. What forever, is the nerve from turn what affirms that vomiting is the psychosomatic expression of the woman who (although she doesn't know it) she really didn't want to get pregnant, and so So the subconscious compels you to vomit in an attempt to reject that unwanted pregnancy. It is nothing more than a crude hoax devoid of everything basis.

Let's not forget that sometimes nausea and vomiting will not have nothing to do with pregnancy but with, for example, gastroenteritis, or let us forget that in severe cases no benefit is observed, but more well it contrary, by losses from weight, dehydration and others imbalances.

In 0.3 to 2 percent of pregnancies, these symptoms lead to a worrying condition called "hyperemesis gravidarum", characterized by the severity from the sickness and from the vomiting, dehydration and lost considerable weight. For all this, do not hesitate to let him be a doctor who will assess your case?

Before from follow, continue go ahead, suits to know what almost all the women successfully complete their pregnancy without requiring any treatment. Just one little patience for the waters to return to their course. They exist in all case, some dietary advice that, although they do not have evidence consistent that guarantee its effectiveness is good to meet.

Avoid the foods copious. Is preferable perform several little intakes throughout the day, without worrying about the fact that alter routines and meal times.

It is the appetite of the pregnant woman that will determine what foods she prefers eat, but it is important to know that foods with a lot of fat (eg: sauces, cheeses, pastries, dairy desserts, fried foods, butter, etc.) usually delay plus weather on Leave the stomach and consequently can worsen the condition.

Avoid smells and textures that cause nausea.

Many women tolerate liquids better than solids, so can try out with prescriptions what soups, creams, juices, Gazpacho, jellies or the like. Some study indicates that acidic liquids or bitters (such as lemonade) are usually better tolerated.

Is habitual prefer the foods cold what hot, because the smell of the latter can increase nausea.

The beverages isotonic 3 (the typical beverages what they take some athletes) they can result tools, on everything Yes the vomiting they are recurring.

No however, the previous advice (I insist, no we're very insurance from that 'work') should not result in the quality of the diet being on the floor (there are women who spend days and days based on cookies salty and ginger ale), because the cure would be worse than the disease.

Without doubt, the support emotional is fundamental. No only the from the couple, who should take care of the house and the food (many pregnant women are so nauseous they can't even go into the kitchen), otherwise as well the from the family, from the friends and from the professionals sanitary. The support of a psychotherapist should not be ruled out, who can help you cope and manage stress. All woman what I carried nail twelve hours without get to hold back none fluid in your body should definitely go to a health center to have it checked. Assess possible dehydration, whose early symptoms are: thirst, mouth dry, pasty tongue, headache, weakness... among others. The doctor, in some cases, will estimate yes is precise Start a treatment for avoid possible complications. One of them consists of vitamin B6 (pyridoxine) what usually combine with a drug antihistamine called "doxylamine", for to block the action from certain substances from our body what they can contribute to the sickness and the vomiting. To the seem, the lack from pyridoxine is involved on these symptom. What any medication, neither is it effective in all cases, nor is it exempt from possible effects secondary and interactions, So what should be used on the dose adequate and always with medical advice. In any case, the Ministry from Health Spanish suggests "to offer treatment with pyridoxine for the relief of nausea and vomiting during the early stages of pregnancy. The recommendation appears in the "Clinical practice guide for care in the pregnancy and puerperium", published in 2014.

I do not find it advisable to "self-prescribe" ginger extracts. The ginger is a plant whose root It is used to treat nausea. It's the only one non-pharmacological treatment recommended by the American College of Obstetrics and Gynecology. Likewise, it is included in its recommendations by the Spanish Society of Family and Community Medicine, although both entities stipulate that the treatment of choice is vitamin B6, alone or with doxylamine. Be what whatever, am supporter from the prudence what Dr. Mingshuang Ding and her team showed in March 2013 at the Women and Birth magazine. They noted that although possibly the extracts of this plant are useful for nausea and vomiting, we do not have sufficient data to evaluate aspects such as: What is the dose from which these extracts are no longer safe?

How long should the treatment last?

What are the consequences of overdosing?

Which they are the possible interactions Come in the extracts from ginger and other medicines or plants?

I would add that food supplements sometimes do not contain what that puts the label and that it is not well evaluated (or agreed) either dose to be prescribed (doses used 4 in different studies range between 600 milligrams/day and 2,500 milligrams/day). The case is what the Research evaluating ginger is promising but not conclusive. We will have to wait for better designed studies. So the things, despite the fact that the consumption of the extracts of this root could help control nausea and vomiting, there is little solid scientific evidence that support, which does not allow to establish a formal recommendation in this regard. This was made clear in an admirable review coordinated by Dr. Anne Matthews and published on March from 2014 on Cochrane Database of Systematic Reviews. His research revised as well the acupuncture, by True, it "showed no significant benefit."

The above considerations are applicable to ginger extracts. Yes, we can safely take ginger in our recipes since the concentration from substances active is a lot less on the food what on the food supplement. Constipation

In pregnancy, the risk of constipation increases due to the pressure it exerts. The uterus (which increases in volume throughout gestation) on the large intestine, along with decreased bowel movements (for absorb plus nutrients from the foods and by effect from the progesterone, a key hormone at this stage). The constipation, what's more from be annoying, it can lead to hemorrhoids. Even more so if the woman performs a lot of effort in defecation. The use of iron supplements, in its case, can contribute to aggravate the frame. The truth is what the pregnant women are no exception: many people suffer from constipation. No is strange, to the view from the amount from foods superfluous what we take (I gave a few examples of superfluous food (see Table 1, in Food in Spain is exemplary (laughs in the background), in the chapter 1).

To diagnose constipation, the professional will take into account that this disorder is defined as the presence of at least two of the following symptoms, during at least a quarter of bowel movements:

Feces lumpy, harsh or what require a high effort for be evacuated.

Feeling of incomplete evacuation.

Sensation of obstruction in the anus or rectum.

Need for manual maneuvers to facilitate defecation.

Less than three bowel movements per week.

Even though no there are tests clear on the effectiveness from the fiber for treat the constipation, on January from 2013, a revision from the Association American from gastroenterology Indian what "the potentials Benefits therapeutic from the fiber dietetics, his under cost, his profile from security and others potentials Benefits for the Health justify assess the fiber (a standard fiber supplement or through the diet) as the first step that should be considered in patients with chronic constipation, particularly in Primary Care". This "first line therapy" means:

Replace the cereals "refined" (bread White, pasta White, flours refined, white rice) for their wholegrain counterparts.

Increase the number from times to the week what we take vegetables (lentils, chickpeas, beans).

Include nuts or dried fruit as snacks.

Drink a minimum from five rations from fruit and vegetables every day.

Reduce the intake of superfluous foods.

All of the above should be accompanied by an increase in physical exercise and an increase in water consumption, according to Dr. Juan C. Vázquez in Clinical Evidence in August 2010. If none of this works, the second option is drugs, after weighing risks and benefits. Pyrosis known What "Reflux gastroesophageal» or "burning", the pyrosis appear when the lower sphincter of the esophagus is unable to hold the juices of the stomach in place, rising into the esophagus, with an unmistakable burning sensation in the sternum area. It usually occurs during late pregnancy and often occurs at night. It is believed that it is not only the effect of the pressure of the fetus on the mother's stomach, but also the hormone progesterone influences on the relaxation the sphincter esophageal lower. The supplements from iron they can aggravate is condition, so what the doctor must assess the appropriate dose in each case.

It is good to know that, despite the large number of pregnant women with heartburn, it is rare for this symptom to lead to serious complications, and it is also usually disappear after delivery.

Surprisingly, there are not many studies on this question. In any case, the consensus documents propose, as a first piece of advice, modify the lifestyle and diet of the pregnant, so I list below some considerations hygienic-dietary:

Avoid foods what can aggravate the symptom what spicy, products acids, citrus, beverages carbonated, chocolate, foods or drinks with caffeine, alcohol (totally discouraged in pregnant women) and high-fat foods, particularly fried foods.

Eat often, avoiding large meals (advice applicable to the whole family).

No smoking (yet another reason...).

No carry garments adjusted, what they can exercise yet plus Pressure on the already weakened sphincter what controls the part higher the stomach.

Do not eat late at night.

No lie just then from eat (expect nail three hours for do it).

Raise the Headboard from the bed some fifteen centimeters. The position horizontal favors the Contact from the fluids stomachic with the sphincter esophageal, it what can compromise yet plus his functionality.

No do exercise during to the less two hours then from eat.

The use from drugs (the "second line from treatment") to times is essential.

RESUME E N

If you have any questions about a pregnant symptom, it is better to see a licensed physician, not a "phytotherapist," not a shaman, holy man, healer, sorcerer, or any of the hundreds of other tricksters.

Nausea and vomiting (which are quite frequent) are related with a higher rate of pregnancy success and a decreased chance of miscarriage, unless they are severe. They normally go away on their own before the 20th week of pregnancy, but there are some ideas and treatments that may help. Any pregnant lady who has been vomiting for more than twelve hours should attend a health clinic. Occasionally, the situation deteriorates into a condition known as hyperemesis gravidarum, which is considered an emergency obstetric condition.

Consuming a diet deficient in fiber predisposes pregnant women to constipation. Consuming more foods of origin, less processed veggies, limiting extraneous items, and increasing physical activity may all assist. After weighing the risks and advantages, the doctor may prescribe specific medications.

Although heartburn is very inconvenient, it is extremely unusual (but not impossible) for it to cause major consequences. There are sanitary and nutritional factors that may help improve the situation, however at times the use of pharmaceutical therapies may be essential.

When anemia has already been formed, a healthy diet will not reverse it; to be more specific, medicines will be used. The therapies are referred to as "alternatives." "have not been shown to be efficacious or safe. Certain dietary advice should be followed.

Although there are few research examining the benefit of lowering salt consumption on pre-eclampsia treatment, it makes sense to consume fewer salty foods, considering that we consume almost double the amount of salt suggested by health authorities. Magnesium sulfate supplements have shown some usefulness in treating this condition, albeit not all research corroborate this. Both the usage of proverbs and the use of medications should be accomplished by discretionary prescription.

Yes, it is critical for pregnant women who have type 1 diabetes to obtain hygienic counseling, preferably from dieticians-nutritionists.

Additionally, it should be given to a woman who suffers from gestational diabetes, which may be averted. Yes, I am aware that they maintain a decent style throughout their lives, that they give the chest, and that they avoid extraneous items such as fast food or "soft beverages." The low-carbohydrate subsistence allowance is not warranted for women with gestational diabetes.

6

Weight gain before to, during, and after pregnancy

Maintaining physical weight is a delicate balance of dedication, renunciations, joys, and exertion. Real pair relationships include ongoing development, conviction, and an active involvement on the part of both parties. Maintaining a healthy weight needs patience and a healthy and active lifestyle, where food is a source of joy rather than pain. THE AURA C AORSI AURA C AORSI AURA C AORSI

There is no need to embark on a diet or pursue a weight-loss plan during pregnancy, since the baby may be harmed? Under no circumstances. What if the expecting mother is obese? None.

What if it's acquiring a significant amount of weight? No, it will not be. What if you are fat and gain a lot of weight in addition to having gestational diabetes? Neither. I begin the chapter with this roundness since it is the most critical of all the points I will discuss below and why, sadly, many women get poor advice on this subject.

However, the period before, during, and after pregnancy are perfect times to begin establishing healthy lifestyle habits, according to people around you. How many of us have strayed from the correct road merely by "What are they going to say"? Prior to pregnancy, you may inform them about the benefits of these preparations for your body, as well as the chances of remaining pregnant successfully (no lie). During pregnancy... well, there is no need for me to provide an explanation at this point; it is self-evident that anything you eat or drink will reach your kid. And after the pregnancy, inform them that «consistent scientific data indicates that if the mother and child father I know eat properly, the chances of his kid making a healthy child are extremely high. Either is a fabrication.

Having said that, I'm going to attempt to reorganize a little bit of what I've learned about weight in these three glorious moments of life. According to his excellent handbook "Control weight before, during, and after pregnancy," the information that surrounds us is "vague, unclear, and conflicting." WEIGHT PRIOR TO GETTING PREGNANT. WHAT IS THE TERM «NORMOWEIGHT»?

This part is critical because, according to the previously referenced NICE recommendation, a woman's weight before to conception "is more crucial in predicting the success of the pregnancy and the health of the future kid than any weight increase during gestation." We know that extreme thinness (which I will explain later) makes ovulation problematic. However, this does not apply to the majority of slender women. Generally, underweight is considered as a risk factor for illness when it is detected only in female smokers (in which case, the goal should be to seek aid to stop smoking) or in those who already have an underlying disease (anorexy nervous, Cancer, AIDS, pathologies cardiovascular, etc.). I discussed it in a piece titled "Am I too thin?" which you may consult by clicking on the following link:

Absent an embargo, Thus, while thinness prior to pregnancy does not necessarily indicate something evil (even though we want thin women to gain weight during pregnancy), it is well established that excess weight can impair fertility (both male and female) and poses a risk to the woman's health and that of the fetus while she is pregnant. Therefore, should they search for women who have "ideal weights" prior to pregnancy? Absolutely. Suits those who have a "regular weight," and those who do not. A normal weight (or "normal weight") ") does not have a finite range of values. I will explain. To determine the weight, we use the so-called "BMI is an abbreviation for "Body Mass Index". To determine this, we divide our weight in kilograms by our height in meters squared (that is, multiplied by itself). If the answer is between 18.5 and 24.9 kilograms per square meter, our weight is normal. I weigh 65 kilograms and stand 1.73 meters tall, hence my BMI is calculated as: 65 kilograms / (1.73 meters x 1.73 meters) = 21.7 kilograms per square meter. I am "normal weight," but what's intriguing is that I would also be "normal weight" if I weighed 55.4 kilos or 74.5 kilos, two distinct values that differ by no less than 19 kilograms. As you can see, the range of what constitutes "normal weight" does not resemble a tiny hole in a golf course, but rather resembles the goal of a soccer field... without a goalkeeper; a good reason to give the red card to anyone who teased me about "weight ideal", "perfect weight", "divine weight of death», or similar entelechies. As Uruguayan writer Eduardo Galeano puts it, perfection is "the dull privilege of the gods."

Yes, our BMI is lower than 16 kilograms per square meter, and we exhibit extreme thinness, which must be assessed by a doctor as well as a dietician-nutritionist, therefore I will not discuss her. If the BMI is equal to or more than 25 kilos/square meters but less than 30 kilos/square meters, we refer to the individual as "overweight." It is prudent to obtain a medical examination to determine your current condition of health. Weight reduction (which should range between 5% and 10% of present weight over about six months) is warranted only if one or more of the following six criteria are met:

You had previously been obese.

I am aware of a youngster whose dads are obese (because our risk from present obesity is higher).

I'm aware that it has gained an additional five kg since last year.

If you are a sedentary person.

Circumference of the waist is more than 102 centimeters (males) or 88 cm (females) (women).

If you have diabetes, abnormal blood lipid levels (such as hypercholesterolemia), or hypertension.

When our BMI is equal to or more than 30 kilos/meter squared, we have "Obesity," and we must immediately see a physician to determine if our extra weight has resulted in any metabolic abnormalities. Additionally, we should lose between 5% and 10% of our present weight in around six months.

We already know what constitutes a healthy weight. And maybe you're now thinking how to lose weight. Thus, similar weight-loss tactics, if any, apply to both pregnant and non-pregnant women, as well as those who already have dice to light, which I mention on the torn apart "To reduce weight before to or after pregnancy. To begin, let us determine how much weight should be won by a pregnant woman.

No, stinging is prohibited. Come during business hours

However, the meals picked must be real foods, not substitutes. A handful of almonds (better if they are not fried or salted), a piece of dried fruit, carrot sticks, or handmade popcorn (without adding salt) are all examples of foods that are good for snacking between meals. At home, we've developed a taste for guacamole, which we serve over bread integral: sandwich, say the cardinals. Reduce the ration by a little amount

Keeping an eye on the piece of the plate or food in front of us is critical if we want to maintain control over the scale's needle's development. In a 2009 declaration signed by three major nutrition associations, he said that "by making minor adjustments to the rations [from the meals ingested], they might reduce energy consumption without stimulating the desire." As an example, reducing the rations will not imply a substantial effort and, as a consequence, it will be able to report effective outcomes in the medium-long term. Both in restaurants and shops (which you should visit with a closed list to avoid succumbing to ultracaloric temptations), the amounts of items vary significantly. They continue to grow in size, which is problematic, since when we have more food in front of us, we consume more without recognizing it.

Olga, who is also my wife, mother, and dietician-nutritionist, had an ice cream a few months ago. I (as an individual) ordered a horchata. To add insult to injury, the temperature dropped 30 degrees and we had walked for more than two hours. Olga requested a cone with an ice cream ball. The clerk stuffed the ball inside the cone and prepared to insert another. "Thank you," Olga remarked graciously, "but I simply want a ball," to which the cashier said, "Yes, but here we placed the second ball free." "Thank you, but I just want one," Olga said, thinking something along the lines of "If my arithmetic is correct, double from balls equals double from calories." "How?" inquired the lady, despite the high cost of listening to an extraterrestrial. I'm telling you that you may take two for the same price." «I appreciate your understanding, but I insist: I only want one." The clerk raised her eyebrows, as if to say, "This aunt is ridiculous," and he handed her the ball. He ran out of tip, and if we did not return, more would have gone missing... To consume, Water

Water is a simple yet vital piece of advise for every postpartum lady. We consume an excessive amount of alcohol, sugary beverages, and juices. Did you know that in the last two decades, the consumption of juices and nectars in Spain has tripled? Sugary drinks, as their name implies, contain a lot of sugar, which raises your risk of cavities and obesity. This also occurs with juices, even homemade ones: fruit sugars are categorized as hydrates of carbon, while the liquids I am familiar with define what are known as free sugars. When it comes to alcohol, keep in mind the WHO message: the less, the better. If you are not taking contraception, abstaining from alcohol is quite convenient. FACTS PRIMARY INFORMATION FROM THE LACTATION MATERNAL

In February 2011, under the direction of Dr. Tony Ogburn, researchers from the universities of New Mexico and Boston studied from cover to cover many obstetrics and gynecology reference books produced since 2003. They did so to ensure that the material they presented on lactation maternal was accurate, up to date, and consistent with current evidence research. They used what reference twenty two in their magnificent work, which was published in the journal Journal of man lactation.

Lactation, which should begin before to the infant's first hour of life and should be administered "on demand," is the most recommended method of feeding a newborn (that is, when the baby wants, and not "every three hours and ten minutes").

The maternal exclusive breastfeeding period (during which the newborn consumes exclusively mother milk) should be prolonged to the baby's first six months of life.

Early artificial milk augmentation exposes the infant and mother to a variety of hazards.

Breastfeeding should continue for at least the first year of a child's life. Baby, and there is no upper age restriction.

Breastfeeding has several advantages for the mother, including less blood loss during delivery, decreased chance of developing breast cancer, emotional benefits, and cost savings.

If you overlooked them, please read them again, since we live in a culture that extols the usage of the feeding bottle, owing to the "powerful gentleman don money." What I'm looking for is something contemporary, scientific, sanitary, nourishing, immunity boosting, and, of course, healthy. The research concluded, as predicted, that the material on mother breastfeeding in obstetrics and gynecology textbooks is inconsistent and often contains significant omissions and mistakes.

That is why I have devoted this brief piece prior to getting started to the nursing woman's diet.

Chapter Six

WHAT BREASTFEEDING DOES TO FOOD AND NUTRIENTS ON WOMEN

What do you juggle if you don't have anything?

Is it necessary for moms to balance their meals like a juggling from the Moscow circus in order for the milk to rise successfully during the puerperium? To be sure, no. AND SO THAT, ONCE BREASTFEEDING IS ESTABLISHED, THE MOTHER PRODUCES NUTRITIVE AND MAGNIFICENT MILK? Neither. To encourage milk production and to maintain breastfeeding, you only need to allow the infant to nurse often during the day and night, or "on demand." Regarding the function of food, below is what the Maternal Lactation Committee of the Spanish Pediatric Association (AEPED) believes:

Except in severe situations of malnutrition, the mother's nutritional state has little effect on her capacity to produce dairy or on the quality of her milk.

In severe situations of malnutrition, we will advise the lactating mother not to give the infant artificial milk. It is preferable to supply the mother with artificial milk (or, much better, with a nutritious diet) in order to maintain lactation.

Numerous ladies have inquired as to whether certain meals affect the flavor of breast milk. The answer is straightforward: no. Not artichokes, asparagus, beans, garlic, or cabbage, nor any other food, alters the flavor of breast milk in such a way that the infant consumes less milk. There are also no foods or substances that "produce more milk," including almonds, sardines, cow's milk, beer, brewer's yeast, wheat germ, or milk thistle. You can verify that I am not exaggerating in the February 2011 issue of Breastfeeding Medicine Magazine.

Water

If you believe that breastfeeding mothers should drink even the vases' water, tea suites read east torn apart.
TO CONTINUE, I will provide two genuine premises and a conclusion, and I will ask you to determine whether or not they are true:

Premise 1: Every day, the woman who bears the chest produces a large amount of milk (truth).

Second premise: the maternal milk is composed of 90% water (truth).

Conclusion: how much plus Water baby the mother will make in addition to milk (is this true?).

What are your thoughts? This conclusion is incorrect. This is referred to as "cheating" logic, a study of what to perceive in a simplistic manner. It seems to be true due to the sea of reasonableness, yet this conceals a fallacy. And it is for this reason that, in order to determine whether or not the statement "The more water the mother drinks, the more milk she produces," is true, we should force a few lactating mothers to drink water in excess of their thirst sensation and compare the amount of milk produced to that of other nursing mothers who should simply drink according to their thirst. To determine the amount of milk extracted by moms, we must weigh them before and after breastfeeding using a reliable scale. will have conducted a comparable experiment? Certainly! Doctor Alex Olsen was the first to do so, publishing his findings in the professional journal Acta Obstetricia et Gynecologica Scandinavica in 1940. "Forced and excessive drinking is neither essential nor useful for nursing, and may even be detrimental," he concluded.

But the confirmation final came up on June from 2014, when the"magazine badge" on the medication based on the evidence, Cochrane Database of Systematic Reviews, released a research whose conclusion was the following:

No there are tests enough what support an intake from liquids plus there from it what is likely what require the mothers babies for cover their wants physiological.

Bottom line: if you breastfeed, drink (water) depending on thirst what have on every instant since neither tea you go to dehydrate by refusing to drink liters and liters of water, nor are you going to create more milk by drinking those «liters and litres."

Energy, proteins, fats and carbs

With relation to energy, like in the case of water, we must not fall into logical traps. Although the body of nursing women requires extra calories, it doesn't even imply you have to eat them all (part of those will come from the woman's fat stores) nor that they have to strive to eat a lot. Appetite is an excellent predictor of how many calories should a nursing lady take in. As for proteins, lipids or carbs, the consumption guidelines are no different in nursing mothers. Supplementation with a particularly trendy form of fat, omega-3s, has not passed the Cochrane screen. The edition from December from 2010 from his magazine included an extensive study led to cape by the doctor Mario F. Delgado-Noguera and their collaborators, what concluded what no there are enough evidence what support the supplementation with Omega 3 long chain in women who breastfeed, to improve growth or the development of their children. Fiber\sConstipation, which affects almost 25 percent of pregnant women, does not disappear in many from they after the Birth, by it what have sense increase the habitual consumption of foods rich in fiber, such as fresh or dried fruit, fruits dry (better what no be fried, and without Salt), vegetables and cereals wholemeal (wholemeal bread, brown rice, wholemeal pasta, etc). (wholemeal bread, brown rice, wholemeal pasta, etc.). In any event, the fiber consumption guidelines are the same in breastfeeding women as in not lactating. Calcium and vitamin D

I include these two nutrients in the same section since they are both important in bone health, as I described in chapter 3. About calcium there would be little bit to say, since the needs from East mineral no rise in breastfeeding (just as they do not in pregnancy), owing to the body absorbs more calcium from food and excretes less calcium via feces and urine.

However, as many people assume what give the chest "wears out the bones", wish let Clear what breast-feed no develops osteoporosis neither puts on risk the Health I mean, such as What verified by the United States Department of Health in 2009, via your Health Research Agency. Actually, we have proof that the longer the nursing duration, the less danger the mother has of experience fractures osteoporotic from hip, vertebrae and extremities superiors. It also, by the way, decreases your chance of breast cancer. Ovary or breast, according to the meta-analyses by Luan and Anothaisintawee that you have in the bibliography.

Nor do vitamin D needs rise at this period. Many cases, I know supplement to the babies breastfed with vitamin D, but this does not justify the mother taking these same supplements (unless presents a deficiency), because, according to the European Safety Authority food, "have few data for estimate from shape precise the increase what I know produces from vitamin D on the milk maternal What response to supplementation with this vitamin by the mother", and There is evidence that transfer of vitamin D into breast milk is restricted. Iron

The guidelines from intake from iron on the breastfeeding they are a lot lower than during pregnancy, and even lower than before the pregnancy. In nursing not only less iron is spent owing to the fact that the body ceases developing a new life, but also because it tends to amenorrhea (the woman stops having her period), particularly if the breastfeeding is "exclusive". That is, the iron requirements for mother on the lactation they may cover up properly with a healthy diet, unless you have iron deficiency anemia (which does not suggest a contraindication to nursing) (which does not imply a contraindication to breastfeeding). Supplements of iron do not enhance the amount of iron contained in breast milk. Vitamin K

Vitamin K supplementation is only justified to increase the amount of this vitamin in the breast milk of those mothers treated with phenobarbital, carbamazepine, or phenytoin, or who have refused what I know manage to the baby newly born vitamin K (the injection intramuscular from is vitamin on the thigh prevents the disease haemorrhagic in neonates—associated pain lessens if the baby suckles during the procedure—).

Iodine

It is crucial that breast milk includes an appropriate quantity of this mineral, because this way the newborn will be able to properly make its hormones thyroid, needed for the healthy development of your brain. It is possible what the professional sanitary tea suggest consume daily 200 micrograms of potassium iodide (pharmaceutical supplement) if you do not eat every day three servings of non-organic dairy products (organic appear to contain much less iodine), plus roughly 2 grams of iodized salt. It's a subject rather contentious, as I have dwelt on in Chapter 3 (Folic Acid and iodine) (Folic Acid and iodine). Without embargo, there existing disagreement some with regard to the need of daily ingesting a pinch of iodized salt, which should not confused with sea salt. It is vital to prevent frequent intake of algae, whose iodine level may greatly exceed safety limits from this mineral. Have more information in the chapter 4. Multivitamins

Yes the multivitamins (what no only they contain vitamins, otherwise as well minerals) are not justified in pregnancy (see other vitamins, others minerals and the Famous (what no reputed) omega-3, on the chapter 3), less yet it is it so on the breastfeeding. No exist testing sufficiently what support their usefulness, and we do have indicators that the continuing use of these preparations may cause a long-term health danger in some persons.

Chapter Seven

RISKS NUTRITIONAL DURING THE LACTATION

Tobacco and alcohol

What the tobacco it impacts badly to the metabolism from various nutrients, I allow myself to label it as a "nutritional danger". I read on the Web the centers for disease Control from state joined what some women they believe what no there are difficulty on return to to smoke a time what the baby is born. The reality is that if someone smokes near the infant or inside house, sure there is a problem: the possibilities of the occurrence of the call "death sudden the lactating", and I know rises considerably the danger of the newborn having lung difficulties. However, if the smoking mother quits nursing, makes a significant error, since the Breastfeeding protects in part from the illnesses induced by passive smoking, while the bottle does not. The benefits of nursing more than surpasses the hazards of the mother maintaining smoking. Even while the milk maternal include anything from nicotine, no contains tar or some components of smoking, very hazardous. And if the nursing lady takes on a nicotine patch to stop smoking, too matches what follow offering the chest to the infant. I insist: the milk maternal from a smoking woman is significantly better for her child's health than any feeding bottle.

And with booze something similar occurs. There is no question that alcohol is always harmful (much more so in pregnancy than in any other stage), but although the deleterious effects of modest exposure to alcohol during the breastfeeding no is it so well documented, Yes it is it so the Risks of artificial feeding. Although alcohol, whatever its kind, is not necessarily healthy (see Annex), breast milk with some alcohol is better for baby health than artificial milk. This is not the case if there is an acute alcohol intake and soon after nursing, since this might induce coma and convulsions in the newborn if breastfed. After a dinner acute from alcohol, I know should anticipate to what the mother east tranquil, on everything Yes the infant is a few weeks old, before nursing. No adult there intoxicated alcohol should practice co-sleeping (sleeping in the same bed) with a baby, since there is a danger of crushing it inadvertently.

The time required to wait to breastfeed so that the alcohol swallowed in an occasional disappearance of milk and blood depends on the weight of the mother (the lower the weight, the more weather) and from the quantity from alcohol taken (to add alcohol, plus weather) (to plus alcohol, plus weather).

Avoid giving the chest till after two and a half hours for every 10-12 g of alcohol consumed: one third (330 ml) of beer, 4.5 percent alcohol; a 120 ml glass of wine, 12 percent alcohol; or a glass of 30-40 ml of liquor, 40-50 percent alcohol. Indicative times to wait for ladies carrying roughly 60 kg weight: a glass from came: 2.5 hours, two thirds from beer: 5 hours, three glasses from liqueur: 7.5 hours, etc.

I remind you that beer does not increase milk production. If you alcohol consumption is high, you should ask for help to deal with this trouble. The consumption of non-alcoholic beer or 0.0 percent is safe in the lactation. Coffee

The coffee hardly reaches the breast milk... although some does. In some children (but not all) irritability, insomnia, tremors or an abnormally high muscle tension (hypertonia) if the mother takes doses greater than 300 milligrams of caffeine per day (see Table 5 in Chapter 7). (see Table 5 in Chapter 7). Some children are more sensitive to caffeine than others, so it is worth each woman values her son's response.

Drugs or Phytotherapy

Other base from data very recommendable, even though on English, is LactMed:

Already I have spoken widely from me opinion on the very popular phytotherapy (see chapters 3 and 8). Here I will only add two considerations. In the first place, that, despite the fact that the risks involved in breastfeeding are notably minors what exist during the pregnancy, these they continue to exist for both mother and baby. I list the herbs classified what from "risk high" or "risk very high" by and- lactation (we found similar results in LactMed):

On second place, his ability from increase the production from milk maternal (by that the they take many women) no is verified on absolute. No it will happen nothing Yes you put on you salad a pinch from some from herbs listed in Table 7, or if you eat a goji berry, but do can happen if you consume extracts from these plants (which have higher concentrations from substances active) or Yes shots to often infusions made with them. Hygiene food

The measures hygienic what I listed on the chapter 4 (Belt from food safety) are valid at any stage of life. Throughout case, as well as certain infections can pose a serious risk for the fetus, the same is not true in lactation: in general, if the mother gets a foodborne infection, it will not affect the production or composition of your milk, nor will it transmit the infection to the baby. Fish and mercury

Although the Spanish Ministry of Health recommended in 2011 that women infants (as well to the pregnant) avoid eat the species plus contaminated with mercury (swordfish, shark, bluefin tuna and pike) 1 , a most recent report of the European Food Safety Authority (EFSA) does not consider it justified for women to "avoid" any fish. The EFSA Yes has indicated what drink plus from three four rations from fish to week may mean ingesting too much mercury, but this applies to the entire adult population, whether or not they are pregnant or lactating. Allergy food

Until make some years, I know advised to the moms from children with high risk of a food allergy (eg, if they already had a sibling with an allergy) who did not take (the mothers) potentially allergenic foods, such as milk, eggs, fish or fruits dry. No however, on December 2010, an extensive and rigorous review published in The Journal of Allergy and Clinical Immunology advised against this measure, as unnecessary. If it is certain what Yes the baby already suffers an allergy food (correctly diagnosed) the mother should not eat the foods to which the child is allergic. Saying this, is important insist on what the lactation maternal protect those children from countless troubles. WHY WHAT CONVENIENT WHAT A WOMAN INFANT EAT HEALTHY?

It is convenient because food plays a fundamental role in health. He does it in all moments of life, but in this case there is three compelling reasons to take a firm grip on the reins of a healthy diet:

1. It will help you slowly regain your previous weight and keep it stable On Spain we're, without doubt, increasing from weight. Practically 6 from every 10 Spanish people have overweight or obesity, so what no we're speaking of a rare disease, but of an epidemic. The point is that after pregnancies there is usually a tipping point in weight body: after several years of stability, in many women it begins to increase inexorably. It is the ideal moment, therefore, to acquire some good ones habits from feeding what allow return, without rush, to the weight previous to the pregnancy and keep it from by lifetime. I have detailed widely different strategies for approach is question on the chapter 6. Exercise, even high-intensity exercise, does not make breast milk less abundant, nutritious or healthy. Weight loss is not a contraindication to breast feeding.

It will influence the feeding of our children (breastfed or not)

The mother's diet influences a little - not much - in the quality of breast milk. We find an example in iodine. If the mother takes salt iodized, his baby will be able manufacture without problems their own hormones thyroid. We also know that the food the mother eats leaves a flavor in your milk, which acts as a "flavor bridge" that facilitates the baby's transition to foods that the mother eats regularly habitual. But the mother's diet will greatly influence something else: how your child will eat over the years. One of the factors that most influences the feeding of our children is the example that we give with our way of feeding ourselves.

Prepare the body for the next pregnancy

A bad feeding decreases your possibilities from success yes you want get pregnant again. Although this is something that also applies to the dad: so much the quality what the amount from sperm from the men who eat poorly is worse than that of those who follow a diet healthy. I explain this because many women, what during the pregnancy have improved their eating habits, after childbirth they resume the previous ones, which were not exactly healthy. In fact, this applies as well to the smoking and to the intake from beverages alcoholic. There are tens of reasons to avoid bad habits and one of them is, as I say, increase the chances of success of a new pregnancy.

9 781804 769607